OIL-PULLING REVOLUTION

The Natural Approach to Dental Care,
Whole-Body Detoxification
and Disease Prevention

DR. MICHELLE COLEMAN

Ulysses Press

Published in the U.S. by
ULYSSES PRESS
P.O. Box 3440
Berkeley, CA 94703
www.ulyssespress.com

ISBN: 978-1-61243-442-1
Library of Congress Control Number 2014952012

10 9 8 7 6 5 4 3 2 1

Printed in Canada by Marquis Book Printing

Acquisitions Editor: Kelly Reed
Managing Editor: Claire Chun
Copyeditor: Renee Rutledge
Proofreader: Lauren Harrison
Front cover design: Rebecca Lown
Cover art: © Olga Lebedeva/shutterstock.com
Interior design: what!design @ whatweb.com
Layout: Jake Flaherty
Indexer: Sayre Van Young

Distributed by Publishers Group West

NOTE TO READERS: This book has been written and published strictly
for informational and educational purposes only. It is not intended to
serve as medical advice or to be any form of medical treatment. You should
always consult your physician before altering or changing any aspect of
your medical treatment and/or undertaking a diet regimen, including the
guidelines as described in this book. Do not stop or change any prescription
medications without the guidance and advice of your physician. Any use of
the information in this book is made on the reader's good judgment after
consulting with his or her physician and is the reader's sole responsibility.
This book is not intended to diagnose or treat any medical condition and is
not a substitute for a physician.

This book is dedicated to all of the amazing doctors I have had the pleasure to know and work with and to all the beautiful people I feel honored to call my patients.

CONTENTS

INTRODUCTION

Every day I am blessed with the pleasure of helping a bustling community in a thriving, affluent neighborhood in the San Francisco Bay Area live healthier and happier lives. My journey studying health has been a long one that started well before I earned a doctor of chiropractic degree in 2005 and advanced to become a platinum level nutrition practitioner in 2013.

As a child I suffered from frequent attacks of bronchitis, colds, and other respiratory illnesses. I never felt better taking traditional Western medicine and even at times suffered side effects that were worse than the reason for taking the medication. My quest to learn about health started when I was 11 years old, when I started reading Dr. Deepak Chopra's works about Ayurvedic medicine and the mind, body, and spirit connection of healing.

I also started to incorporate proactive steps into my own life, like regular exercise and positive mental affirmations that made a huge shift in improving my health. I saw a chiropractor for checkups and learned that the brain and spinal cord communicate to every part of the body via the nerves. This greatly improved my health in many ways, one being a dramatic decrease in lung-related sicknesses.

Small changes to my diet made a huge impact on how I felt as well. In college I studied about the human body for a full 10 years; however, even into my doctorate program I kept reading about the mind, body, and spirit connection in Ayurvedic medicine. It was very real to me that all of these factors matter. I noticed that the weekly practices of yoga, Pilates, prayer, and walking greatly enhanced my energy. Shifting to a heavily plant-based, organic diet gave me even more energy. As time went on, I kept seeing my chiropractor then added an acupuncturist and holistic dentist to my team of health leaders.

Oil Pulling and Wellness

I started studying the work of Dr. Weston A. Price five years ago when I decided to expand the level of nutritional counseling services we offered in our clinic. Dr. Price was a dentist who had traveled the world and made profound discoveries in the field of nutrition and health. He went to remote societies and figured out that they have better health than more industrialized nations do, and that evidence of this is in their gleaming white teeth. He discovered that eating real foods and incorporating vegetables, animal fats, and protein are necessary to strengthen the health of each generation. Sugar, processed wheat, and manufactured starches are most certainly things that tear the body down, starting with oral health then traveling through the entire body. He found that people with diseased teeth subsequently have diseased bodies.

As a result of Dr. Price's influence I began eating a primarily vegetable and meat diet, incorporating some fruits and whole grains and lots of healthy fats. On this diet, I noticed the biggest leap in health I had ever experienced. The cold I would get a few times a year lessened in severity and duration and, at times, I would go almost a whole year without getting sick. Not yet sure of its full benefits, I added occasional oil pulling to my wellness regime. My dentist remarked that I could do my cleanings only once a year and, even then, there was hardly anything to clean. This is when my oil-pulling research really started.

Inspired by a seminar headed by Dr. Freddie Ulan, a well-known chiropractor and nutritionist out of Florida, whose work is frequently studied by many in my field, I had already been reading studies on different fats and how they affect the body. Dr. Ulan's advice had been to use oils on scars to keep them from blocking the body's energy flow.

Experience had shown me that certain oils used on the body do in fact help scar tissue on the skin to heal. At my wellness clinic, the acupuncturist and I often recommended the use of oil on certain scars for one to two months, after which our patients saw huge improvements in health. One patient started using sesame seed oil daily on a scar under her chin, and after 30 days she was sleeping better and suffered less from symptoms of hypothyroidism .

After reading article after article on sesame oil's benefits to heart patients, I turned my attention to my own father, who has a long history of root canals. He was eventually diagnosed with type 2 diabetes and heart disease. While there were some dietary reasons, including too much refined sugar, wheat, and processed dairy consumption that had led to the diabetes, the heart disease was a mystery to the doctors. There was zero family history of heart disease, and his diet had already been greatly improved at the time of the heart attack and subsequent heart disease diagnosis. I ran into PubMed articles about heart patients all having one common thing in common: a history of root canals or gum disease. In this book, we'll explore the undeniable connection between oral health and the body.

Dr. Weston A. Price was the pioneer that led me to this understanding. Dr. Deepak Chopra had led me to Ayurvedic medicine, which frequently applies fats to the body in a manner similar to what I had been doing under Dr. Freddie Ulan's advice to keep the meridians flowing.

After finding that fats are equally important to oral health, I started oil pulling, or gargling with oil, and recommended my family and patients do the same. Here are some examples of how it's helped them:

- My dad had a flare-up of an old dental problem, so I gave him coconut oil, cinnamon, and clove. After oil pulling for a few days, his pain disappeared and his inflammation came down. I encouraged him to keep pulling for 20 minutes daily.

- A former patient had osteonecrosis of the jaw, or destruction of the jaw via an autoimmune condition in the body. This was the result or side effect of using an osteoporosis drug many years before. I had her start oil pulling with coconut oil and a few drops of lemon oil. After a few days she, too, noticed the destruction slowing down and started to experience more comfort in her mouth.

- For a pregnant patient with persistent nausea and gum soreness, pulling with coconut oil made her gums feel better in a week and greatly improved nausea symptoms.

My own teeth are smoother and I received compliments of whiter teeth after only one week of oil pulling. I really noticed a difference when I let my practice of oil pulling fall by the wayside at a time I was busy running a business and planning a wedding. In desperation with seasonal sinus flare-up, I pulled out my coconut oil with a drop of peppermint and oil pulled for 20 minutes. My sinuses cleared up instantly and it lasted all day.

I have found that, like anything in life, you just have to make it a priority when you start something new. Being a chiropractor and nutritionist for a decade now and seeing amazing benefits with my patients approaching health proactively, I know you do not have to suffer through life piling on more conditions as you age. You can reverse your age and regain and preserve your health. Your body can thrive. I know this—I feel better than my 16-year-old self at just a bit over double that age. If someone asks me if they should oil pull, I say absolutely! There is no reason not to. You will ONLY see benefits. The worst-case scenario is you will not see or feel benefits because you are already so healthy! If that is the case, congratulations, and keep doing all of the things you are doing to stay healthy and symptom-free! My advice is to find the time each day to take care of yourself. As I tell all of my patients, YOU are worth it.

CHAPTER 1

WHAT IS OIL PULLING AND WHERE DID IT COME FROM?

In a life full of hustle and bustle, wouldn't you want to maximize your dollars and time with a simple new habit that could dramatically improve your health? It is hard to believe that something so very basic and affordable could yield such amazing health benefits, but it does!

Oil pulling sounds mysterious—most people have never even heard of it. Yet it has been around for thousands of years, longer than current fields of traditional medicine and dentistry. It is a valuable lost art among today's bargain jugs of mouthwash, fancy teeth-whitening agents, electric toothbrushes, and miracle liver cleanses. Its benefits far outweigh the time and financial investment involved.

What if I told you that for 5 to 20 minutes and 25¢ or less a day, you could dramatically improve your oral health, save on dental bills, have a brighter and whiter set of pearly whites, and experience a cleaner, healthier body with more energy and less pain?! Would you try my amazing suggestion? Well, you may even have a jar or bottle of the appropriate oil sitting in your house. All you need is the proper information to get started.

A Lost Art

Before we get down to business and detail the what, why, and how of oil pulling, let's explore where this ancient art began. The roots of oil pulling lie in Ayurvedic medicine. Ayurveda is an art of living in daily balance with the laws of nature. Its ultimate goal is not only to heal a diseased person, but also to keep the healthy person healthy.

The word "Ayurveda" is a Sanskrit term meaning "science of life." "Ayu" means "life," or "daily living," and "veda" is "knowing." Ayurveda was first recorded in the worlds' oldest literature, the *Vedas*. Oil pulling is mentioned in the Ayurvedic text *Charaka Samhita*, in which it is referred to as "kavala graha" or "kavala gandusha." The book attributes it with curing many diseases, such as migraines, diabetes, tension headaches, asthma, and more.

Considered today to be alternative and even by some people, esoteric, Ayurveda has been around for about 5,000 years. It has been practiced in daily life in India since its onset, much longer than current-day Western medical practices have been, and is considered to be the starting place or mother of all medicine. Ayurveda recognizes that in order to have success and attain one's true purpose on earth, one must have good health and experience the most out of life with the body they have been given. The Ayurvedic approach includes daily routines that support the body and prevent diseases from occurring. Many of the approaches of medicine today, especially in the Western world, focus on waiting until a disease has manifested itself in the body in the form of symptoms. Ayurvedic medicine primarily approaches health from a preventative standpoint, something that is growing in popularity in the informational age where people have decided they want to live well. Ayurveda strives to help people be their best and thrive, as each life has a purpose. Poor health, whether mental, physical, or spiritual, can inhibit a person from carrying out their life purpose.

Western medicine treats everyone like they should be the same. Ayurvedic medicine recognizes we are all different and while our bodies may need some of the same things to be healthy, our needs vary individually.

Ayurveda recognizes that from the moment we are conceived, we have an individual constitution created by the universal energies of air, water, fire, earth, and ether. A perfect balanced state is one in which the body's three fundamental energies, or doshas (vata, pitta, and kapha), are in balance. The five elements create the three doshas.

Vata is the energy of movement and is made up of air and ether, pitta is the energy of metabolism or digestion and made up of fire and water, and kapha is the energy of structure and lubrication and made up of water and earth.

In order to maintain optimal health, one must determine their primary dosha or doshas and keep them in balance.

This balancing act requires personal responsibility and action. If one is aware of what is shifting in their body, they can make appropriate, proactive choices and remain in a healthy state. It is also important that the body, mind, and soul, which are in constant movement and interaction, be in balance. Systems such as yoga, meditation, rest, relaxation, aromatherapy, meditation, breathing exercises, nutrition, lifestyle, medicinal herbs, cleansing, and physical exercise address this on a daily basis and affect healing.

In the Ayurvedic system of medicine, oil pulling is considered something that helps keep the doshas in balance. It's referenced in the original texts with the use of sesame oil. Sesame oil has been used in many different ways in the Ayurvedic system, most of them related to cleansing and detoxification. The benefits of ingesting sesame oil have long been studied and include decreased inflammation and cardiovascular benefits. High in vitamin E, sesame oil has also been touted for its ability to heal new and old scars optimally. Even though it is not ingested during oil pulling, it is no surprise that an oil with such amazing health benefits was chosen.

Modern-Day Rebirth of Oil Pulling

Oil pulling was mentioned in Ayurvedic texts as oil "swishing" or "oil gargling." It wasn't until the 1990s that it was renamed and presented as "oil pulling" for the benefits we know of now.

Dr. Fedor Karach, a Ukrainian physician, brought oil pulling to the attention of scientists and doctors at an oncology conference in Ukraine in 1992. At the time, Dr. Karach had a compelling reason to share this information. He personally experienced being rid of chronic blood disease and arthritis with daily oil pulling. He explained the benefits of pulling toxins from the body, thusly ridding it of chronic diseases. He even presented the information that in old traditional Indian writings, the human body was said to last for 150 years with 20 minutes of oil swishing per day! He advocated the use of sunflower oil, as it was historically used in India. Many doctors questioned Dr. Karach on the controversial body of information he presented. His article, however, was still published in 1992 in a medical publication. This was the beginning of the modern-day spread of the technique, even leading to its being repopularized in India, where it had still been used by some.

In 1996, a study published in the South Indian newspaper *Andhra Jyoti* documented that oil pulling helped 89 percent of people surveyed be cured of one or more diseases. The survey included the details of 72 miscellaneous cases, 56 blood sugar–related cases, 74 heart and circulation cases, 91 joint cases, 21 hormone cases, 137 elimination cases, 155 digestive system cases, 171 skin cases, 191 respiratory cases, and 758 cases of pains in the body.

What Is Oil Pulling?

Oil pulling is essentially using oil as a mouthwash or oral rinse. In this process, however, so much more than good breath and clean, healthy teeth is accomplished. Choose an oil, such as sunflower, sesame, or coconut. Other oils can be used, but those are the most popular. The chosen oil is then swished around the mouth for 5 to 20 minutes. Training yourself to pull for 20 minutes in the morning is the optimal practice (details to be discussed in Chapter 2), but starting with 5 minutes and working your way up is recommended.

The oil is swished about the mouth, teeth, and gums, causing bacteria to adhere to the oil, suffocate, then dissolve into it. Every single bacterium is covered by a fatty lipid layer surrounding it. This is a fatty protection that keeps it safe, similar to the double-layered fatty membrane or lining surrounding the cells inside our bodies. The fat in the membrane or layer around the bacteria are drawn toward the fat in the oil, causing the bacteria to be drawn out from the oral cavity.

Numerous studies published in medical publications have proven a decrease in *Streptococcus mutans*, the main bacteria that causes dental decay, as a result of oil pulling. Not only are bacteria that cause plaque, decay, and bad breath rid from the mouth, the detoxification system is activated, causing the body to begin flushing harmful substances, such as heavy metals and chemicals, from the body. The other thing that occurs with oil pulling is the decrease of inflammation in the gums and oral cavity. All oils that are traditionally used for this process have been linked to decreasing inflammation. Oil pulling, or swishing, as it was known in the past, is recommended as a frequent activity to maintain proper oral hygiene.

CHAPTER 2
HOW TO OIL PULL

Oil pulling is actually a quite simple and inexpensive daily habit to work into your life. The process of oil pulling starts with taking approximately a tablespoon of oil into your mouth and swirling it around for 5 to 20 minutes. Fifteen to 20 minutes is the optimal duration to pull, but it is recommended that beginners start with 5 minutes then work their way up to 20 minutes, increasing the amount of time they pull each day. If you have a smaller mouth, you may want to reduce the amount of oil to whatever is tolerable, possibly even down to a teaspoon or less. You can eventually work your way to higher amounts of oil once you become more comfortable with oil pulling and know what amount works for you.

To oil pull, swirl the oil around the front and back of the mouth, over the tongue, and toward the back of the throat without swallowing. To maximize dental health, it is recommended to pull the oil in and out from between the teeth and around the gums as well.

To maximize the benefits, there are a few things you can do to prepare your mouth before you pull.

- **Floss and use a tongue scraper.** Start by flossing the teeth and running a tongue scraper over the tongue. You may want to take note if there is a coating on your tongue. A coating on the tongue can indicate toxins in the small intestine, large intestine, or stomach. For many years, the health of the tongue has been used in Chinese medicine as a hint of what is happening in the body and for clues as to whether the digestive tract and organs of detoxification are doing what they are supposed to be doing. Acupuncturists have looked at their patients' tongues at every visit for centuries to note the health of the patient. If there is a very thick coating when you first wake up, you will want to scrape this off to remove oral bacteria, or candida, so that the oil does not get stuck trying to clean up the tongue coating for the whole 20 minutes. By flossing the teeth and scraping the tongue, you will actually be allowing the oil to reach deeper areas of the mouth so that it may do its job in between teeth, into the gum lines, and even into the beginning of the throat.

- **Incorporate probiotics**. Probiotics are healthy bacteria that we need in our diets for our intestines to function normally. The foods you can find them in are kombucha (a fermented tea drink you can make or find in most health food stores), yogurt, Kefir (a fermented yogurt drink also found in health food stores), sauerkraut, miso soup, tempeh (fermented soy beans), dark chocolate, and some pickled foods.

- **Drink water**. Another thing you can do is to drink a glass of water before you oil pull. While there is mixed information out there on how traditional this is, many practitioners, including me, recognize the need for hydration when detoxifying. My only warning is to make sure that doing so does not make you nauseated. Some people have very sensitive tummies, and the water before swishing might aggravate it. The only way to know is to try drinking water before oil pulling and see how you feel.

- **Eat later**. Most writings about this ancient art discuss doing oil pulling first thing in the morning before eating any food. Oil pulling is best done on an empty stomach because some people have reported feeling nauseated while oil pulling. The movement of the mouth imitates mastication (chewing) while swishing and actually signals the body that you are eating. Even though there is no food in your mouth, your liver and gallbladder will respond and can produce bile, and your digestive system starts to work while you swish. This process actually assists in the detoxification of the body while pulling. However, if you have a full stomach, you do not want the experience of it emptying due to the oil pulling initiating that! Although oil pulling is best done in the mornings to avoid any potential nausea you may experience, it can also be done later in the day. When you're first starting out, try all times of the day and see which one feels and works best in your life.

When and where should you oil pull? You can do it while you're sitting at a desk reading emails, taking a shower, doing a crossword puzzle, playing a game on your phone, cooking breakfast for the family, or watering the garden. The main thing to remember is you will not be able to talk for 20 minutes, so go somewhere conducive to a quiet state.

Please note, you do not want to ingest the oil. As we talked about before, the oil kills off viruses and bacteria and pulls harmful toxins into it. These are not things that you want to ingest. The best plan is to swish the oil around your mouth, along the gums, and in between your teeth, then spit it out.

Plan ahead to be near a trashcan or a place where it will be acceptable to spit the oil out when needed. You do not want to spit the oil down a sink or a toilet. The oil is carrying toxins and waste products that should be discarded in the trash. Also, you may end up clogging the drain with an oil such as coconut oil, which changes form and solidifies at different temperatures.

If you need to speak, sneeze, or otherwise open your mouth, spit out the oil that is in your mouth and start over. When you spit the oil out, note what it looks like. The oil that starts out clear will often take on a cloudy or milky appearance. This is good news because that milky appearance is caused by dead bacteria and toxins that have been pulled into the oil. When you see that milky substance, you absolutely know that something has been pulled into the oil to be discarded.

If you are someone who gags easily, you may feel like you are gagging at times. If this is severe enough, spit some of the oil out. This could be a sign you are using too much to start with! You can also spit all of the oil out and just do smaller sessions of 5 to 10 minutes until your body gets used to pulling.

Oftentimes while pulling, people will start to get a mucus formation in the mouth and/or down the back of the throat. If you find this uncomfortable then you may spit out the oil and start with a new batch to keep the benefits going. Twenty minutes of swishing adequately suffocates and kills any bacteria in the mouth. While oil pulling is best done in one continuous session, it can also be broken down into shorter, back-to-back sessions if needed.

After oil pulling, it is recommended to swish or gargle with warm saltwater to rinse the oral cavity. This helps to ease any inflammation and heal any microtears or abrasions in the gums. It also allows for any stray bacteria or toxins left behind to be removed from the body. After swishing you can then brush your teeth with or without toothpaste to finish off the clean feeling.

Oil pulling should be practiced for at least 30 days or one full month before it is evaluated for its true benefits. Many people report benefits after about four days of pulling. Teeth are whiter and smoother, and breath improves!

Step-by-Step Oil-Pulling Guide

1. Use a tongue scraper to remove any excess debris from the tongue.

2. Use floss to remove any debris from in between the teeth.

3. Choose between coconut, sesame, or sunflower oil to pull with.

4. Choose an essential oil you would like to add to the base oil, making sure it's an essential oil you can use orally. (This step is optional but beneficial. See page 71 for more information on essential oils.)

5. Prepare a tablespoon or less of the base oil with one or two drops of any essential oil you are adding.

6. Make sure you are near a trashcan or other appropriate place to spit out the oil. As an alternative, grab a cup if you will be sitting far away from those locations.

7. Put the oil in your mouth and start swishing!

8. Pull the oil in and out from between your teeth and around your gums, but make sure not to swallow it.

9. Swish the oil continuously for 5 to 20 minutes, depending on your comfort level. Beginners may start at 5 minutes and work their way up to 20 minutes, which is the ultimate daily goal!

10. At the end of your oil pulling session, spit the oil into a cup or trashcan. Note the color—a milky-white color indicates success at collecting and ridding your body of toxins and bacteria!

11. Sprinkle a dash of sea salt into warm water and gargle with it to clean out any stray bacteria or residue.

12. Brush your teeth for a few minutes with or without toothpaste to clean off any stuck particles.

Oil-Pulling Chews

A neat and tidy way to oil pull is to make an oil-pulling chew. These great little packages are not actually chewy but are very handy! To make them, take coconut oil (the only oil you can make these with) and place the desired amount for pulling in a silicone mold. You can find these online or in the kitchen aisle/department at the stores, as they are used for ice trays. Silicone molds are often made in fun shapes like hearts, Christmas trees, pumpkins, or just plain circles or squares. After you have placed a tablespoon or so of oil into the mold, you may add an essential oil if you'd like by placing a drop or two into the coconut oil. Mix the essential oil into the coconut then throw your molds into the freezer.

After an hour or less, your oil-pulling chews should be solid in shape. You can take them out of the mold and store them in the freezer in whatever container you like. Having the chews handy makes pulling very easy as you just run over to your freezer and pop a chew into your mouth! As it slowly melts into your mouth, you are ready to start pulling. This is a great option for those of you on the go in the mornings. Moms driving the kids to school can grab one on the way out the door and pop it in their mouth after dropping the kids off. The drive home is a quiet and ideal time to start the pulling routine. Or, run to the kitchen in your robe to grab a chew first thing in the morning, then hit the shower for cleansing and pulling.

This option avoids your accumulating any bottles of oil in your bathroom and gets rid of the random spoon-in-your-bathroom problem too!

While in transit the chew should not melt as long as it is not out at a warm temperature for too long; in colder climates or seasons, it is totally safe.

Frequently Asked Questions

Do I need to oil pull every day?

Optimally you would oil pull every day, just as you brush your teeth every day. Oil pulling for 20 minutes a day is the optimal target to achieve. I have seen people experience benefits from oil pulling four times a week at 20 minutes, but it will take you longer to achieve your goals this way.

When will I see benefits?

Right away you will notice some benefits! Within days, smoother and cleaner teeth and better-smelling breath are commonly reported. Teeth whitening really depends on the color or hue of your teeth, but people have reported a difference in a week and certainly within one month. The healing of diseases can take longer and really depends on your body and how long the ailments have been present. I usually recommend three months for healing results of chronic conditions, as it is a truly slow and gentle way to detox.

Do you oil pull before brushing your teeth?

Yes! You are bringing all the bacteria out to play. If you brush before oil pulling it will not hurt you, but you will need to brush again after.

Do I still need to brush and floss?

Yes! You may not need to use toothpaste or harsh mouthwashes anymore, but the physical action of brushing and flossing is still recommended to help remove any food or debris particles stuck around the base of the teeth and gums. Plus, dry brushing places stress on the gums, a good exercise to keep them stronger!

When is the best time to oil pull?

In the morning after a glass of water, before you have eaten. If you are a swing shift or night shift worker, then after you have slept and before you eat. This is the optimal time to be on an empty tummy. If you miss your morning window you can wait till a meal has digested, about three hours after eating to be safe. Some people like to do it before bed. Just make sure your dinner is long gone so you don't upset your tummy in any way!

Can you oil pull more than once a day?

No more than twice a day is recommended for oil pulling. Traditional references recommend one time

HEALING CRISIS

A healing crisis is when the body experiences symptoms from the healing process. This occurs during detoxification programs and in many other healing arts. Symptoms from oil pulling tend to be mild, the most common being a mild sore throat, mucus formation, or post-nasal drip.

You may also feel flu symptoms, or like you are getting sick. This can be the body's response to old toxins being released. It will not be a strong reaction but can make you feel suboptimal for a little while. Sometimes, when certain toxins are released, like medications, you may begin to feel the physical or psychological effects of the medications, similar to those that occurred when you were taking them.

Healing crisis symptoms could also consist of those associated with the conditions you are healing from. Occasional gas, bloating, and nausea can occur with people who have had exposure to many toxins or medical drugs, or even with people healing from food-related gastrointestinal conditions. The reactions, again, are generally very mild and pass quickly. However, the severity varies from person to person. The sicker you have been through life, the more likely your reactions may be stronger.

If this happens, do not stop pulling. See a health care practitioner to make sure a reaction that concerns you is not caused by something other than a mild healing crisis.

in the morning, but for people with serious dental problems to resolve, twice a day is recommended. In that case, oil pull one time in the morning before eating and three hours after dinner before bed the second time.

How does it taste once bacteria is pulled into the oil?

Most people do not report a change in flavor. It does, however, start to feel thicker as you pull things into it. The flavor of the oil will dissipate or lessen in strength after pulling for a while.

Are there side effects?

There is always the potential for hitting rough spots. Any person with a chronic disease such as ulcerative colitis, Crohn's disease, psoriatic arthritis, rheumatoid arthritis, Hashimoto's thyroiditis, Addison's disease, MS, Parkinson's disease, chronic migraines, gallstones, chronic sinusitis, and many more should realize that sometimes the body can go through a healing crisis.

Oil pulling is a very gentle way to cleanse the body and most people report very few to no side effects. If you have a long-standing condition, however, and have done very little detoxification in the past, you may experience more symptoms than others do. It would be best to support the oil-pulling lifestyle with proactive activities like staying hydrated (page 96), daily exercise (page 100), and maintaining a healthy diet (page 97).

CHAPTER 3
DENTAL HEALTH

Since the time you were little, you've been told to visit the dentist, brush, and floss to keep your teeth healthy. Have you ever wondered why this is important or known what else you could do for oral health? Your mouth actually tells you a lot about what is going on with your overall health. It can also contribute to very serious health problems if it is not well cared for. That's why the journey of health begins in the mouth.

Connection between Oral Health and Body Health

Greek physician Hippocrates believed that all diseases could be handled by focusing on the mouth. He would pull a diseased tooth in order to cure someone from a body riddled with arthritis. Dr. Weston A. Price contributed a lot of research to this topic. Some of his better-known studies link the potential toxicity of root canals to autoimmune diseases like multiple sclerosis.

In his research to prove that bacteria-ridden teeth are a problem to overall health, Dr. Price implanted clean teeth (clean from the exterior) under the skin of rabbits. After a few days the rabbits reportedly suffered from the same health problems, ranging from heart disease to arthritis, of the people whom the teeth had been removed from. The teeth caused the diseases to remain in the body!

Dr. Price was a huge advocate of eating a very clean and nourishing diet of real foods. It was obvious that oil pulling would only add to that, maintaining the health of the oral cavity by pulling the bacteria in the teeth and gums out of hiding and ridding them from the body.

Oral Bacteria

There are hundreds of bacteria and sometimes more in your mouth at any specific moment. And there are over a million that actually will exist in your mouth over time! I am sure you have heard somewhere that the mouth is the dirtiest place on the body. In many ways, this is true.

Bacteria are routinely found in our food and even in our water supply in trace amounts. Think about sharing drinks, food, and kisses with people or even animals! Each time this happens we pick up new microscopic friends and leave some microscopic friends behind to share. Our bodies contains more foreign critter DNA than human DNA. A lot of what is in our bodies is actually good, or friendly, bacteria. The problem comes when we pick up unfriendly or bad bacteria or if the amount of good bacteria is so vast that the body has a hard time managing it. At this point, it can do damage to our body. *Streptococcus mutans*, the not-so-friendly bacteria that causes cavities, is at the top of the list of unfriendly bacteria.

Cavities

The most well-publicized dental health problem, cavities are something we hear about from childhood, complete with fear tactics that stress brushing as a way to avoid them. The fear of pain has always been an effective way to motivate people into heeding advice from a doctor! We have all heard a story about going to the dentist and getting the dreaded drill used on our teeth to fix a serious problem.

A cavity is tooth decay caused by bacteria. The bacteria eats away at the tooth, creating a hole. If the hole gets big enough, it can compromise the health of the tooth. The tooth can cause pain and may eventually require drilling, filling, or in severe cases, extraction. Eating sugary and starchy foods can definitely contribute to bacteria in the mouth growing and creating a sticky adherence to the teeth and gum line; it then proliferates, leading to more downstream problems.

Gingivitis

Gingivitis, or gum disease, is another frequently talked-about oral health issue often discussed on TV ads selling oral hygiene–related products. This is a condition where the gingiva or gums become infected and inflamed due to bacteria that causes plaque buildup. Plaque is a hard substance that is created at the gum line and on the tooth in response to bacteria, mineral salts, and saliva combining. The buildup irritates the gums, causing them pain, swelling, and inflammation. The gums will appear puffy and red and feel irritated and sore. Gingivitis left on its own to get worse causes the gums to bleed and pull away from the tooth.

Bacteria in the Bloodstream

When pockets of bacteria become really infected, a chronic inflammatory response is triggered and the body can turn on itself, attacking its own tissues and bone and eating away at the foundation the tooth sits in. A serious issue arises when the bacteria travel down tiny pathways in the gum line into the bloodstream or heart. For many years, across medical disciplines, it has been known that serious dental procedures like root canals are correlated to heart disease. Bacteria released into the bloodstream from the mouth to the heart is a much more serious problem than cavities, although both can be avoided with proper oral hygiene.

Abscesses

Another unpleasant consequence of bacteria in the mouth is an abscess. An abscess is a pus (dead bacteria)–filled pocket at the base of the tooth created by an acute infection of a tooth. The main symptom reported is a very painful and throbbing tooth. The infected tooth is usually sensitive to heat, cold, and pressure. Eventually, if left untreated, the symptoms progress to swelling of the face, jaw, neck, and lymph nodes surrounding the area. A fever may develop. In time, an abscess may rupture, leaving a foul taste in the mouth. If left untreated, the infection will often travel to other parts of the body, as referenced above. Infections left to progress untreated lead to periodontitis, where the connection between the teeth, gums, and jawbone is broken down. When the ligaments that hold your teeth to your jawbone are disrupted, there is no anchor to hold them in place. The symptoms of this problem are actually quite mild, at first, and quickly progress. By the time most people know they have a problem, it is far too late in the process to avoid surgical intervention.

Pockets in the gums can form, allowing food and bacteria deep within. The bacteria can then eat away at the bone and root of the tooth. Gum disease is very serious in that it can produce loss of teeth and painfully diseased gums that need surgical removal. Advanced surgical procedures caused by this process can be quite costly and are often not covered by insurance plans.

Halitosis

A less serious yet bothersome oral hygiene issue is halitosis, commonly known as bad breath. This is something most people would like to avoid. Bacteria or fungus-like candida cause a stinky environment in the mouth. I remember my mom saying to lick the back of my hand from time to time throughout the day and smell it after a few minutes. If it was stinky, I needed to brush my teeth again! Such an exercise offers a glimpse of mouth odor. Many times, people are unaware of their own scent wafting out of their mouths.

Oil pulling is very well-known for helping to get rid of this problem. The essential oils chapter (page 71) recommends which oils are best to add if you encounter this scenario.

Color of Teeth

Another less-worrisome thing relating to oral health is the color or hue of the teeth. Many people enjoy drinking coffee or soda, or eating foods that may stain their teeth. Smoking is also something that will discolor or darken one's teeth. Many expensive dental products on the market use chemicals to whiten your teeth. As with oil pulling, these products usually require a daily time investment. The difference is they are more expensive, use chemicals, and offer no additional health benefits. Oil pulling offers many potential health benefits and if other essential oils are added, the benefits increase.

One of the most amazing benefits of oil pulling is not having to use mouthwash anymore. You should always continue to floss while oil pulling, as it helps the oil get in between the teeth. Should you still see a dentist for periodic checkups? Absolutely! Will it decrease the frequency of visits and increase time between cleanings? Yes it will! And it will make life for your dentist easier with fewer projects to work on. This accounts for an overall cost and time savings to you.

Pregnancy and Dental Health

During pregnancy, many women are focused on what they eat and the things they put into their body, like medications. They do not realize that the health of their unborn child is also affected by their dental health. Studies prove that oral health during pregnancy creates a healthier baby and less chance for preterm labor or low birth weight.

An important note for pregnant mamas is that the bacteria in your mouth, good or bad, can enter into the amniotic fluid. If any harmful bacteria does cross into this sacred space, the baby could be in harm's way or at risk for complications. To keep this from happening, pregnant women should eat a diet low in starchy or sweet foods. Natural fruit sugars are not a problem, but foods high in white sugar or processed carbohydrates, like muffins, cakes, bagels, and pastries, could cause problems to arise. Eating real, fresh, whole foods and including healthy bacteria in fermented foods such as yogurt and sauerkraut is great. Brushing, flossing, and oil pulling help the gums as well. There are very few ways that a pregnant mom can safely detox while pregnant. Oil pulling is one of them.

You should make sure that the oil being used is safe for pregnancy. Sesame oil and coconut oil are both fine, and many essential oils are safe to add.

A number of moms report oil pulling as helpful for morning sickness. One of the main reasons is it supports the action of making bile from the liver and gallbladder, hence improving digestion, an area where a lot of pregnant women struggle. Where for some people it can cause nausea, for many pregnant women oil pulling actually stimulates digestion and calms the nausea response. This is, of course, up to the individual. Expectant mothers should start with 5 minutes first and see how that makes her feel. If she finds it helpful it is a wonderfully safe way to remove toxins from the body, especially the mouth, keeping a safe environment for mama and baby! In some rare cases people will experience more extreme detox reactions like headache and nausea. If this occurs, it would be best to wait until after pregnancy to resume oil pulling. Also, if you gag easily, pregnancy is likely not an optimal time to oil pull as the gag reflex can be exacerbated.

Oil pulling provides a way to keep the mouth hygienic. By keeping the mouth clean you will maintain healthy gums and prevent cavities. Oil pulling eats away at all of the bad-breath-causing bacteria and cleans the surface of the teeth, which makes them whiter! You can handle almost all dental health concerns by oil pulling.

CHAPTER 4

HEALTH CONDITIONS BENEFITED BY OIL PULLING

A collection of health conditions have been reported over time to be helped by oil pulling. By keeping oral hygiene in check with oil pulling, you also benefit the entire body.

Cardiovascular Diseases

Almost every single person walking around with heart disease has a history of a root canal or other serious gum infection. If a heart condition exists, a well-known danger is developing bacterial endocarditis, a bacterial infection of the inner surface of the heart that creates inflammation and further cardiac health problems and complications within a few weeks of a dental procedure. This is why many dentists require certain patients to take antibiotics, even for procedures as simple as a dental cleaning.

The biggest concern with heart disease is plaque buildup. We already know the Standard American Diet, or "SAD," leads to plaque via sugar and white flour. We also know that unmanaged diabetes can create arterial plaque due to the buildup caused by starchy and sugary foods and unmanaged blood sugar in the vessels. Now, studies show that certain bacteria that are present in arterial plaque are the same bacteria found in the oral cavity. This is starting to prove the theory of bacteria migrating from the tiny capillaries in the gums to the vessels of the heart and the body.

Studies show that sesame oil is very healthy for heart patients. A 2013 study published in the *Journal of Cardiovascular Disease Research* concluded that "chronic administration of sesame oil offers cardio protective action via putative antioxidant property." Such studies focus on ingesting the oils, but as we know, a certain amount of the oil will be absorbed into the body while oil pulling. Very high vitamin E content makes this oil a great one for daily use with heart patients, as it helps to oxygenate the body. It also has high antioxidant value, which is very healing and preventative for a heart patient.

Of course a healthy diet of real, unprocessed foods is recommended. But taking extra measures to keep the oral cavity clear of bacteria can help a heart patient stay well and keep a non-heart patient from becoming one. If you have a history of heart disease in your family, oil pulling with sesame oil would be a very proactive thing to start doing.

Inflammation and Osteoporosis

One of the most common health issues is inflammation. Inflammation occurs in response to disease or injury. The body produces inflammatory mediators called cytokines. The cytokines are your immune system's answer to boosting the inflammatory process, and they are necessary. However, a problem can arise when we have inflammation near a bone or near teeth. Cytokines can lead to bone destruction and reabsorption, which in turn leads to the loss of bone density. The loss of bone density is called osteoporosis. Osteoporosis, over time, creates a weakness in the bone, leaving it vulnerable to fracture. The jaw is the most vulnerable place for this activity to occur. If the bone breaks down in the jaw, it is easier for bacteria and inflammation to spread throughout the body. This, in turn, creates more cytokines and more inflammation. This is how chronic infections and chronic inflammation develop. This cycle is the reason why herbs or homeopathic medicines that are supposed to decrease inflammation are also immune boosting.

Oil pulling can help stop this degenerative process from occurring. The best oils to use to maximize benefits for decreasing inflammation and preventing osteoporosis are sesame oil and coconut oil.

Gastrointestinal Diseases

This is one of the fastest-growing areas of dysfunction and disease today. Health practitioners see more and more people with IBS, ulcers, Crohn's disease, ulcerative colitis, food allergies, food sensitivities, and just plain malabsorption problems. Gastrointestinal health is directly impacted by the health of the oral cavity. The bacteria in the mouth are ingested into the stomach and the cascade of effects from there take their toll on the pancreas, liver, gallbladder, and small and large intestines.

Daily stress can wear down the body's normal activities in relation to stomach acid and enzymes. When one ingests a food, normally the HCL, or hydrochloric acid, in the stomach begins to break it down, including the bacteria. We know that stress can overproduce or underproduce acid in response. Usually the body underproduces. The result of this is a rotten and acid feeling in the stomach. This is very often misdiagnosed and people are mistakenly given antacids. If an antacid is given to someone with low acid, ironically they might feel better because it neutralizes part of the rotting response. The problem is the bacteria that were in the food and mouth now pass on through to the rest of the digestive tract. Long-term, these acid-blocking patients begin to have other digestive problems due to bacteria that can now pass freely from the mouth or from any foods in the entire digestive tract.

H. pylori is a well-known opportunist bacteria often hanging out at the gum line. It can easily pass from the mouth to the stomach, causing stomach ulcers. Stress and antacids are the biggest culprits leading to an H. pylori ulcer.

As a result of ingesting the "SAD" foods, one of the main problems today is inflammation. While eating these foods the body kicks up inflammatory and even autoimmune responses. Oil pulling can greatly decrease inflammation in the mouth and stop the bacteria from causing any additional problems downstream.

The body can use all of the help it can get naturally. This leads to less need for more invasive medical intervention.

Lung Diseases

In the colder months, lung and bronchial infections are very common in many areas. There are several different reasons for this. An interesting yet overlooked fact is the change in diet during a seasonal change. In colder temperatures, people tend to go for starchier and sweeter comfort foods. This leads the teeth and body to be at more risk healthwise. It is not commonly known that people who have no teeth are not riddled with as many lung diseases as those with teeth! Since extracting everyone's teeth is not the best option, we'd better learn how to keep the oral cavity and teeth as healthy as possible.

Just as a heart condition can be triggered by oral health problems, a lung disease can be set in motion by a dental infection. Many of the very serious lung diseases seen in hospitals today are caused by bacteria normally found in the oral cavity. What happens is these bacteria feed on the unhealthy sugars and starches in the oral cavity and then overpower and outgrow the normal flora balance in the mouth. Everyone has choked a bit on their own saliva right? Doesn't it always makes you feel silly? The bigger problem is this can happen any day and even at night when you don't know it! Now if your immune system is very strong and you have a normal flora bacteria balance in your mouth, you are not at any risk of developing a lung infection. However, if you have been eating processed foods, are stressed, are over middle age, have any other immune-compromised state, have a history of alcoholism, diabetes, or smoking, you are at risk of developing a lung infection from the bacteria living in your mouth! By having poor oral hygiene and aspirating the improper flora you can cause yourself a lung infection. Eating whole unprocessed foods, avoiding starches and sugars, and oil pulling daily can help you avoid laying in the hospital with pneumonia or being down with bronchitis.

Oil pulling helps to clear the sinus passages, leading to less mucus pouring down the throat and into the lungs. Oftentimes while pulling, people will have to stop and start over due to the immense amount of cleansing that can happen in this area. People will cough, sneeze, snort, and spit out secretions that the body is expelling due to bacteria and toxins being drawn into the oil. This leaves a healthier, clearer respiratory tract.

Skin Conditions

Did you know that your skin is an outward reflection of how toxic your system is? Your body will push toxins out wherever it can—this includes the skin. A doctor of Chinese medicine can look at your face and tell you what organ system is toxic, diseased, or struggling by the pattern of acne on your face. Oil pulling not only provides nourishing oils with anti-inflammatory properties and immune-boosting capacity close to your face, it also gets rid of toxic residues from viruses, bacteria, and fungi that have been residing in the skin. In case studies, the conditions that have been helped by oil pulling are acne, wrinkles, eczema, psoriasis, and rosacea. Overall quality of the skin has been reported to improve, especially the brightness!

The only side note, as referenced before, is the possibility that once the oil pulling has started, it can kick up a healing crisis (page 33) or detox reaction. This can create some serious upset for someone trying to clear a face that now looks worse. Don't stop if this happens. Instead, drink lemon water for a healthy antioxidant boost, eat clean, and follow the other guidelines in this book. It means you have hit the jackpot on just what your body needs. For some people it will get worse for a while before it gets better.

Many people report tension of the skin improving, fine wrinkles and lines disappearing, looking younger, and improved overall look. Even dark circles have been noted to disappear.

Sinus Congestion

One of the most prevalent conditions I see in practice is chronic sinus congestion. Many times it is seasonal, but it can also be from dietary or detox-based causes. The body will create excess mucus in the sinus area in response to allergens, pollens, and dust in the air. It can also be a response to the level of toxins in the system. Someone with a more toxic load in the body will tend to have more sinus congestion. The other potential cause is food allergies. Some patients have varying degrees of food allergies. Increased sinus congestion while eating certain foods can indicate a sensitivity or allergy to that food. Dairy is one of the main problem foods that causes a sinus problem. Oftentimes switching to raw or grass-fed milk, goat or sheep's milk, or raw or grass-fed cheeses can help. If none of these seems to improve things, trying almond milk and giving the body a dairy break can provide relief. If you love the taste of butter but find it also causes you congestion, you can use an Ayurvedic substitute, ghee, which is clarified butter. Many Indian-based companies that sell ghee will sell a "cultured ghee." This means most of the milk fat has been removed. If dairy is not the problem, gluten may be the culprit (those are the two most common sinus allergy–related foods). If not, then move on to cleansing. Eating a diet of mostly animals, plants, whole grains, and fruits can help eliminate a lot of trigger foods. There is a very in-depth cleansing ritual in Indian culture that happens with seasonal changes. It involves using oil on the body and in the body to cleanse.

Oil pulling not only helps the mouth stay healthy, which is valuable due to the proximity to the sinuses, but can pull toxins into the oil and reduce the body's burden during seasonal or climate changes.

Do your sinuses flare when you travel? Again, oil pulling with some coconut oil and a drop of lemon and peppermint can instantly clear up the sinuses and help ease the burden of processing new allergens or pollens.

In Chinese medicine an overburdened liver will create sinus congestion. I put people on a 21-day cleanse program of whole real foods and high doses of whole food veggies and see clear sinuses as one of the main reported benefits!

Chronic Fatigue

Chronic fatigue is a new diagnosis that's shown up in high number in the last few decades. Many times it results from doctors testing everything under the sun and not being able to find a diagnosis. There can be an underlying adrenal fatigue issue that is oftentimes missed in the world of Western medicine. The number one thing I hear from people who come into our clinic is having increased energy after a few days or weeks on our program. When you start to focus on restoring the normal functioning to the body and you feed it real foods and detoxify the system, it is able to function without the burdens of toxicity and lack of energy flow.

Oil pulling can reduce your toxic load and decrease the number of pathogens or unfriendly bacteria, fungi, and viruses that your body has to deal with on a daily basis. This can greatly enhance the amount of energy left for other activities and can help you get out of a chronically exhausted state.

Insomnia

Insomnia is an extremely common problem for people of all ages. The reasons for it are vast and challenging to spot. I have had great success putting people on a whole foods diet, cutting out processed foods, and being very strict about sugar consumption. Again, the benefits of detoxification ring loud for this problem too! My patients have reported sleeping better after launching into a 21-day detoxification program. After one week of oil pulling, people report getting better-quality rest. It really comes down to the fact that in the evening when we sleep the body goes through a systematic protocol of cleansing and restoring the organs. If someone keeps waking up in the middle of the night, it usually means an organ system is struggling to function properly. It is literally a wake-up call that it needs help. By starting an oil-pulling regime you can affect the entire body, taking stress off the organs so that they may function more effectively.

Arthritis

Recently, doctors have discovered a connection between diet and every type of arthritis. We know that for osteoarthritis (the most common form), red meat and processed flours and sugars increase the rate of spreading and severity to the body. We know that nightshades are bad for psoriatic and rheumatoid arthritis. And we know that viruses, bacteria, fungi, and toxins cause more inflammation and aggravate all forms of arthritis. This, again, makes a huge case for a whole foods diet with careful attention to learning which foods aggravate the condition. It also makes a case for oil pulling. Reducing the inflammation, toxic load, and immune system threats greatly helps the body to thrive.

Autoimmune Conditions

This is another category becoming more common today in patients of all ages. With autoimmune conditions, the body uses its defenses against itself. Not enough is known in this area in the Western medical world and the best treatment today is to use medications that suppress the immune system's ability to function. Such drug ads are more and more prevalent on TV, and listening to the list of side effects is depressing. The problem, as you can imagine, with a medication that suppresses the body's immune system is vulnerability to attacks by viruses, bacteria, and fungi. These patients are the most challenged with getting a solid footing on a cure. Figuring out a special whole foods diet that omits any inflammatory foods or potential allergies or sensitivities is the cornerstone, followed by a healing regime. Oil pulling will gently pull toxins, which is so necessary for these patients. The bonus of killing off viruses, bacteria, and fungi will help support the system of someone who is autoimmune-challenged.

Indigestion

Based on the number of people carrying Tums with them on a regular basis, it is obvious that indigestion is a pretty common problem. Multiple factors are at play here. Yes, choosing plenty of whole foods and fewer processed foods is a great start! There is more to the picture, though. Gas, bloating, belching, and even stomach pain are common signs that the body has a chemical toxicity.

By oil pulling, you actually stimulate digestion and help cleanse the body at the same time. You also reduce that potential immune invader load that could contribute to infections and problems down the digestive line.

General Health and Detoxification

Oil pulling can pretty much help any condition. Why? Because, as we have well explored in detail, your oral health greatly impacts the entire body—negatively or positively. The body needs help detoxifying. An analogy I use daily is when I opened my new wellness clinic a few years ago, we brought in an electrician to evaluate our space. We were installing an x-ray unit and it was an older building, so we had to evaluate what we needed to do to make it work. He gently explained that with the building's limited energy, we needed to put in a special x-ray unit that would conserve energy using batteries so that we did not drain the building and cause mini blackouts whenever we took x-rays. I relate this to the body's organ systems. We only have so much energy to run our bodies. If something like a toxin, virus, bacteria, or fungus diverts energy away, it is hard for the body to function normally.

In today's world we have created billions of toxins in order to maintain modern-day life. The fetus of today is exposed to more chemicals before birth (via the mother) than ever. A study published by the Environmental Working Group in July 2005 found 287 chemicals in umbilical cord blood passed from mother to baby. These chemicals were from everyday sources like non-stick cookware, plastics, pesticides, flame retardants, packaging on fast foods, and air pollutants. We produce toxins at an alarming rate and the scary part is they are also in our food and water. According to the WebMD article "Drugs in Our Drinking Water," a study done in municipal water districts looked at water quality in 24 major metropolitan US cities and found trace amounts of varying drugs in every single water supply. Even though there are only trace amounts, the article does cite that the Potomac River and other rivers have seen male and female fish take on opposite-sex characteristics due to hormones in the water supply building up in the fish over time. So even while eating as cleanly as we can, we drink and bathe in toxins and they build up and are stored in our fat cells.

Rather than using this as doom-and-gloom news, I say it's a wonderful thing that we have information to share on these topics. You can exercise and eat clean to support the body and add oil pulling to your daily or weekly regime. You will see some benefits soon after starting. Smoother, cleaner, whiter teeth are guaranteed! And if you do suffer from health problems, they may take some time to heal. Since each person is different, it is hard to say exactly how long. The main thing is to keep your eyes and mind on a healthier, more energetic you. Start a journal of your results! This way, you can share it with others.

CHAPTER 5

THE OIL-PULLING OILS

First of all, why use oil at all? What is so great about oil compared to mouthwash? Why not just use lemon water? Well, these are very good questions and actually quite easy to explain. As briefly mentioned before, the lipid membrane layer that surrounds a bacterial wall is repelled by water. Water is neither attracting nor threatening to a bacteria in any way. Bacteria is, however, very attracted to another oil because of its fatty covering. The bacteria just emulsifies into the oil you are oil pulling with. It gets drawn into it and suffocated. This is why the oil turns a milky-white color when you are pulling. That milky-white color is evidence that bacteria has found the oil and become one with it! Brushing, flossing, and seeing the dentist for checkups are always great habits to have. Oil pulling regularly should be added to keep the bacteria in your mouth in check and make all of your other habits for oral hygiene and overall health more effective!

CHOOSING THE PROPER OIL

It is really important to choose high-quality oils. If you cannot afford or do not have access to cold pressed and organic oils, use the best you can get your hands on. It will still work for detoxification, no matter what vegetable oil you use, but its health benefits when absorbed may not be as high. You are always going to absorb a certain percentage of the oil into your body, so you want to use very high quality when possible. The best oils to use are:

Organic extra virgin coconut oil, unrefined

Organic cold pressed sesame oil, untoasted

Organic cold pressed sunflower oil, unrefined

You can use other oils such as organic extra virgin olive oil or organic peanut oil; however, there is not as much information present about the health benefits of these oils when oil pulling. The most commonly used oils in India are sunflower and sesame oil. In recent times, coconut oil has become very popular, especially in the West.

Coconut Oil

Coconut oil is an edible oil made from coconut meat from the coconut fruit. It is high in saturated fat, which makes it very stable and less likely to go rancid. A jar can last a few years with no spoilage!

South Asian and tropical cultures have traditionally used it in their cooking for many years. It has a very high smoke point, meaning it is a stable oil to sauté and fry with. The oil stays available for your body to use, even when exposed to high temperatures. Some oils change when you cook them at high temperatures, and this inhibits you from using them for baking and or frying foods. This makes coconut oil an optimal choice for cooking.

In Samoa, coconut oil has been used to soothe the teething process of infants for centuries. In the West, Sri Lanka, and South India, people prefer to utilize coconut oil for oil pulling. This could due to its pleasant and mild taste or its growing popularity in the diet.

In recent years, the use of coconut oil has flourished in many cultures, especially in the West. You will find tons of recipes on the Internet and in popular, current-day cookbooks that contain coconut oil due to its health benefits and high smoke point. You will also find it used in multiple ways for health. It is used to heal skin conditions such as psoriasis, eczema, chronic dry skin, acne, and stretch marks. It is used to quench dry hair and is said to have weight-loss benefits when ingested regularly. Coconut oil, when consumed, is used for energy by the body. The body will not store it, but is rather efficient about using it as a resource to burn as fuel.

As you may be familiar with, coconut oil is solid at colder temperatures and turns liquid as room temperature increases. You do not need to heat the oil before using it. Just take a small chunk out of the jar and put it in your mouth. Within seconds, the heat of your body will warm it to a liquid, the perfect state for oil pulling.

Coconut oil stimulates blood flow and has high amounts of vitamins E and K, great vitamins for heart health and the body's healing process. Coconut oil contains a large percentage of lauric acid, which increases HDL (high-density lipoprotein) and LDL (low-density lipoprotein) levels in the blood, creating an overall better cholesterol profile due to raising "good cholesterol."

Many homemade, cost-effective skin regimes involve coconut oil, from using it in your hair for cleansing and conditioning to using it as a regular deeply hydrating lotion to using it on a cotton ball to remove makeup. It can also be used for making a homemade shaving cream when whipped together with other oils like shea butter and essential oils and placed in a glass jar. With its versatility of uses, every person should have coconut oil around the house. This makes it easy to have around for oil pulling too!

Coconut oil contains a medium chain fatty acid that plays a major role in detoxifying the body. It is antifungal and antibacterial. It has the potential to kill viruses that have a lipid or fatty coating on them. Most viruses and bacteria have a lipid coating on them. *Streptococcus mutans,* the bacteria responsible for tooth decay, E. coli, the bacteria responsible for urinary tract infections, and streptococci, found in many sore-throat related infections, are killed by coconut oil. Candida is also killed by coconut oil. A white-coated tongue can be a sign of thrush or oral candidiasis, a fungal infection. This can, however, be resolved with oil pulling and diet change, where coconut oil would be your oil of choice!

Prior to 1954, when rumors of its saturated fat content started to circulate, coconut oil was known to be the most nutritious oil, with numerous health benefits. When people started to misunderstand the oil, doctors and nutritionists discouraged people from using it. Today, people who are more traditional or old school in their thinking will continue to dispense the same old information that coconut oil is bad for you. The plain and simple truth is, it is not bad for you unless you have an allergy or sensitivity to coconut. Many current-day studies have completely debunked any myths that once existed about coconut oil.

Sesame Oil

Sesame oil is an edible oil made from pressed sesame seeds. Sesame oil is one of the primary oils used for EVERYTHING in South India, from cooking to cleansing the body to oil pulling. It is the oil of choice for many health-related uses in Ayurvedic medicine, one them being to rid the body of heat and restore balance. It is used in oil lamps kept in the shrines for Hindu deities. It is also used in South Indian temple shrines.

Sesame oil is touted for the high antioxidant factor contained in sesamin. It is high in vitamins E and K and polyunsaturated fatty acids, which make it great for healing. It also has antibacterial properties, though it does not get as much popular press for this quality. One important side note for heart and high cholesterol patients is that sesame oil is helpful for having such high antioxidants that it absorbs bad cholesterol from the liver.

Many practitioners today use sesame oil topically to handle the healing of scars and for those employing Chinese medicine principles, to unblock stuck chi.

Sesame oil is actually a fairly stable oil but can still benefit from limited exposure to light and heat. Storage in an amber bottle and refrigeration are best. Limited exposure to air is recommended, too, so replace the lid once the amount you need is poured. Buy smaller bottles and use sesame oil frequently to maximize the benefits.

Sesame oil is a lightly flavored nutty and palatable oil. It is not hard to talk people into using it. It is easier to use because it is liquid and does not need to melt and can easily be poured onto a spoon and into your mouth. It is a great oil to cook with because it has a very high smoke point, like coconut oil. It is actually the preferred oil for use in frying tempura in Japan.

Many studies discuss the overwhelming benefit to heart patients of ingesting this oil. Due to the healing nature of its antioxidants and high vitamin E profile, which improves oxygen to the heart, it is the oil of choice for people with heart conditions or those trying to prevent a heart condition. It is ingested for the purpose of lowering bad cholesterol and a study published in the January 2015 issue of the *Journal of Medicinal Food* shows it is effective for such. Research also shows that it acts as a gentle antifungal, making it a good candidate for someone with fungal issues, or candidiasis, as evidenced by a September 2013 study published in the *Biological Research for Nursing Journal*.

Sunflower Oil

Sunflower oil is made from pressed sunflower seeds. The roots of this oil date back to the 1800s in Russia, where it has traditionally been used in the food and cosmetics industries. It is mostly a mix of monounsaturated and polyunsaturated fats, oleic acid (omega 9), and linoleic acid (omega 6), with a small amount of stearic and palmitic acid. Because it is made of these oil blends, it is less shelf-stable and very susceptible to oxidation and rancidity and should only be stored in amber bottles in a dark, cool place. It is also easily degraded by heat, which makes it suboptimal oil to cook with. It is, however, fine to use at the oil-pulling temperature of the body.

The only controversial thing about sunflower oil is its high amount of omega 6 fatty acids. You want to have a one to one ratio in the body of omega 3 to omega 6. By consuming too much omega 6, you can potentially increase inflammation. If you have plenty of fish oil or flaxseed in your diet to balance it, this is of a lesser concern. You also are only going to absorb a fraction of the oil as you pull, since you are not ingesting it.

A NOTE ON QUALITY

The thing about oils is quality matters. Evaluate the oil before buying a jug from a discount warehouse store. Is the oil stored in plastic? Plastic degrades and can actually leach into the oil you are using. Glass storage is optimal. How long has it been on the shelf? Check the dates on your oils! While some oils, like coconut oil, are shelf-stable for many years, you still want to know how old your oil is and not let it expire as it can go rancid.

CHAPTER 6
ESSENTIAL OILS

Anyone who has studied essential oils found organically occurring in nature knows that we were clearly meant to use them as medicine. Essential oils have been around for centuries, with their earliest usage to cure human ailments recorded in biblical times, predating any current-day medical or pharmaceutical approach by far. As a matter of fact, the various active ingredients used in many current-day medicines mimic the action of an essential oil.

Oils have been used topically, aromatically, and internally for desired health effects ranging from digestive support, antiaging, and improved energy to antibacterial properties, antiviral qualities, and cancer prevention.

There are quite a few essential oils worth discussing that can be added to the base pulling oil (sesame, coconut, or sunflower) by adding a drop to the spoon. In so doing, you can enhance the effect or provide an added benefit to this 20-minute investment of your day. For pennies on the dollar you can add a few drops of any of these oils! The thing to note about pulling is that your body will absorb some of the oil, so quality matters. Interestingly, once toxins are expelled by pulling and brought into the oil, they will not reabsorb into the body, so it is a win-win. You absorb all the good stuff and get rid of the bad!

The first thing to note is whether it is an essential oil that you can safely ingest. The bottle will clearly state if it is safe for you to ingest or if it is safe for oral or internal usage. In order to add it to your oil-pulling regimen, just put your base oil on a spoon, then add a few drops of the essential oil to the base oil. If you are using multiple oils, then add one to two drops of each essential oil you have selected. Remember, this mixture will be in your mouth for about 20 minutes, so the more drops, the stronger the flavor. Make sure the essential oils you use to pull are organic or therapeutic-grade oils to ensure the quality of what you are exposing your body to while pulling.

Basil Oil

Basil oil can assist those with abdominal or digestive distress accompanied by migraine. Basil has long been studied for its digestive and body elimination support. Many cultures include basil in their food, which makes sense since it assists with digestion and is a natural antibacterial, keeping food clean. Many migraines start with problems with the liver and gallbladder. A migraine that involves digestive upset most often is connected with those two organs needing support.

Basil is an herby and spicy scent, has a mentally uplifting effect, and promotes mental clarity. It is an invigorating oil to wake you up in the morning. It blends well with quite a few oils, from citrus-based oils to lavender, and will blend well with any base oil.

Bergamot Oil

Bergamot is a wonderful oil with a sweet, citrusy, and refreshing scent. It is known for its analgesic, anti-inflammatory, antiseptic, and mood-lifting qualities. Bergamot is a very good grounding oil for emotional distress. Its neuroprotective quality has been studied and demonstrated in brain injury cases (AromaTools 2014). From an oral health perspective, it has shown to be effective at helping cold sores resolve. It has also demonstrated to be effective at resolving thrush, an oral candidiasis infection. It blends well with lavender and lemon and any base oil.

Cinnamon Oil

An essential oil that is best known in its dry spice form is cinnamon. Cinnamon oil is also used in the field of oral health and hygiene. It is known for antibacterial, antiviral, anti-inflammatory, antiseptic, antioxidant, and immune-boosting benefits.

Cinnamon oil has the amazing ability to enhance the effects of any oil it is paired with. It has been used in Ayurveda for healing benefits in cooking. It has a warm, sweet, and spicy aroma that is well noticed during the holiday season and in teas and baked goods. It is also great for helping balance blood sugar in that it supports the pancreas. This oil fights viral and bacterial infections. According to the fifth edition of *Modern Essentials: A Contemporary Guide to the Therapeutic Use of Essential Oils*, after testing, there has yet to be a virus, bacteria, or fungus that can survive its presence. It is best blended with clove oil and orange oil and blends well with any of the base oils due to its strength of flavor.

From the Ayurvedic perspective, this oil is good to use during the colder or damper seasons, as it promotes warmth and circulation. It can also be used to assist the body when headache and sinus congestion are present. Cinnamon oil has a calming and grounding effect emotionally. If you can handle the spiciness of it, this would be an overall great oil to add to your pulling regimen. Some people may be sensitive to the warmth of this spicy oil; make sure to only use one drop to the tablespoon or so of the base oil. This oil is not recommended during pregnancy.

Clove Oil

An essential oil long understood as powerful for oral usage is clove oil. Clove oil is primarily used for analgesic, antibacterial, antiviral, antifungal, disinfectant, anti-oxidant, anti-inflammatory, antiparasitic, and strong antiseptic purposes. It is a general immune stimulant. Many cultures use clove oil on the gums of teething babies to lessen discomfort and provide an antiseptic environment. One study shows a strong antifungal effect on candida strains. Another study shows clove oil to reduce the production of alpha-toxin, enterotoxin A, and the *Staphylococcus aureus* bacteria. Yet another study shows clove oil to have an antibacterial effect on several respiratory pathogens, which is important with oil pulling because the mouth can harbor immune challenges to the respiratory area due to proximity.

Clove oil is one of the oldest-referenced oils in Ayurveda and is used in many cooking recipes. It is most famously found today in chai tea. It has a strong and robust aroma, and one drop goes a long way. A good combination consists of a drop of clove, cinnamon, and orange oil to coconut oil for an immune-boosting combination reminiscent of chai tea.

Clove oil can be applied directly to gums by applying one drop to your finger and rubbing on the gums in the case of a toothache. To oil pull, combine one drop of it with a base oil of choice to a spoon, then swish for pulling purposes. The Chinese traditionally used clove oil for bad breath. It is a very strong oil, however, so it may be wise to put one drop on the spoon and let the base oil diffuse the flavor. It is all up to tolerance and preference, but both methods of direct application or swishing will get the job done of helping a toothache and providing better breath!

Fennel Oil

A great oil for digestive support is fennel, which specifically helps the liver. Fennel is also known to support the pancreas with blood sugar balance and clear tissues of toxins. It has a sweet and spicy aroma and flavor with licorice undertones. It blends well with peppermint, ginger, lemon, and lavender. It will blend well with any base oil.

Ginger Oil

A great oil to use while pulling if you tend to get a bit queasy or experience any digestive upset is ginger oil. It has a lovely sweet, spicy, and woodsy scent. It is known for its antiseptic properties and support of the digestive tract. Ginger demonstrates results similar to an antiemetic drug, thus decreasing nausea (AromaTools 2014). Ginger has also been used historically to prevent scurvy, an oral disease.

Another use for ginger in Chinese medicine and Ayurveda is warming the joints to lessen the effects of arthritis and joint pain. Ginger has been noted to lessen the pain from a sore throat. It blends well with any base oil and pairs with the essential oils of citrus or spices, such as clove and cinnamon.

Grapefruit Oil

Fruity and upbeat, grapefruit oil is another great day starter. It has a clean and fresh, yet bitter scent and flavor. Grapefruits have been promoted for their liver, kidney, lymphatic, and vascular cleansing benefits. It is well-known for antiseptic, disinfectant, and mood-lifting benefits as well! Its antioxidant levels assist the body in a preventative manner, as with other citrus oils such as lemon and orange.

A really wonderful benefit is that grapefruit oil supports the adrenal glands. These are the little glands responsible for regulating stress and providing us with consistent energy throughout the day. So while it enhances the detoxification effect of oil pulling, it also gives your body a boost. It blends well with peppermint and citrus and any base oil.

Lavender Oil

Lavender is a wonderfully healing and balancing oil with floral notes and sweet undertones. There are so many uses for lavender, one of the most well-known and documented being its calming effect on anxiety and insomnia. It is also known as an antifungal, anti-microbial, anti-inflammatory, analgesic, antihistamine, and antitoxic agent. Lavender can be used to help heal oral herpes or any other oral inflammation. It blends well with citrus essential oils and any base oil. If oil pulling makes you feel anxious or if you want a calming, grounding 20 minutes, this might be your oil to add. This oil should be heavily diluted during pregnancy and not used orally.

Lemon Oil

A simple yet very powerful addition to your base oil is lemon oil. The benefits of lemons for their detoxifying nature has been known and promoted for years throughout nutritional education and alternative medicine circles. Lemon oil is also an antiseptic, antifungal, antioxidant, and antiviral agent. A few drops of pure, undiluted lemon oil can contain the oil of approximately 60 lemon rinds, depending on the brand. Lemon oil has a bright and uplifting aroma and has been known to positively affect mood. It is very cleansing and will assist the liver in removing impurities from the system. A great bonus is that lemon oil is generally one of the most inexpensive oils to purchase. Lemon oil has a very pleasant, fruity, and mild taste. It blends best with coconut oil from a flavor perspective, but can also blend with sesame or sunflower oil.

Melissa (Lemon Balm) Oil

A rare and expensive oil that can very effectively be used to heal cold and canker sores is Melissa oil, or lemon balm. Melissa oil demonstrates inhibition of herpes simplex type 1 and 2 (AromaTools 2014). It is best known for antibacterial, antihistamine, antimicrobial, antiviral, and antidepressant effects. Historically Melissa oil was used for nervous disorders and to promote fertility. It was the main ingredient in Carmelite water distilled in France since 1611 by the Carmelite Monks. If using Melissa to help a canker or cold sore, it is best done with shorter oil pulls of 5 to 10 minutes, three times a day. The frequency is needed to quickly remedy the problem. It has a delicate lemony scent and blends well with lavender, floral, and citrus oils. It will blend with any base oil for pulling.

Myrrh Oil

A less-talked-about essential oil that goes all the way back to biblical times is myrrh. One of the very wonderful things about myrrh is it works very well to help scars heal. It would be the perfect oil to use for receding gums, gingivitis, or to assist the healing process after dental surgery or oral injury of any sort. Myrrh has been found to reduce interleukin (chemicals believed to play a role in inflammation in the gums) (AromaTools 2014). This oil can help increase appetite if someone is struggling to have one. It is also good for fungal infections, so an oral candidiasis infection would respond well to it. It is used on oral ulcers to aid healing. It is a very strong oil; one drop per pull is all that is recommended.

Orange Oil

Unique uplifting and calming benefits are reason enough to add orange oil to your oil pulling routine. Orange oil has been used for years in popular cleaning products for its antiseptic benefits. It has also been used to assist the body with any digestive upset related to nervous stomach.

Orange oil blends well with other citrus oils like lemon and grapefruit for enhanced cleansing and antioxidant benefits. It also blends well with the clove and cinnamon oils for an immune-boosting trio.

Oregano Oil

This oil is not for the faint of heart. It is a very strong oil that is antifungal and immune-boosting. It blends well with any oil because it is so strong it will overpower whatever oil you place it in. It is a very good oil to use during flu season, when the body can really use a boost. One to two drops maximum is all that is needed. This oil should not be used during pregnancy.

Peppermint Oil

Everybody loves a minty fresh mouth! Peppermint oil is a favorite essential oil for oral health. It is commonly added to natural toothpastes and mouthwashes. Pure

A NOTE ON PREGNANT WOMEN AND KIDS

Many oils are safe for children and pregnant women, especially when they are diluted in a base oil, but it is best to check with a health care practitioner or purchase a guide to know for certain. There are many places online to buy books with details about essential oils and their usage. I recommend AromaTools.com for a solid guide on overall usage. Any oils I recommend for pregnancy specifically are safe, as are all of the base oils.

peppermint oil has many benefits beyond its lovely, refreshing scent. It is best known for digestive support. Peppermint is also used for calming a nervous stomach, helping to quell nausea, and calming dyspepsia. Peppermint has a bright and lively aroma that has been touted for its mood-lifting effect and improving alertness. Great to add to a morning oil-pulling ritual, it will help to wake you up!

Peppermint is also traditionally used to help stop headaches. It is used to alleviate sinus congestion and is very effective at assisting the opening of blocked nasal passages. It has such a strong aroma it overpowers and can blend well with any main pulling oil.

This oil should not be used orally during pregnancy.

Tea Tree (Melaleuca) Oil

One of the best-known oils used in face washes, shampoos, and multiple natural remedies is melaleuca, or tea tree oil. It's best used for antifungal and antibacterial purposes, as noted in multiple studies. This oil is very strong in odor and flavor. Even one drop may be challenging to stomach for too long in oil pulling. It is, however, one of the strongest and most documented oils from a success rate standpoint. It is a very good oil for canker and cold sores. Tea tree oil has been shown to inhibit the herpes simplex virus (AromaTools 2014), the virus responsible for canker and cold sores.

Tea tree oil has also traditionally been used to prevent periodontal disease and would be a great oil to add for gum problems.

Oil Combinations

There are a few combinations of oils that are worth mentioning for different desired health benefits while pulling. The oils can be blended evenly in an amber glass bottle, then a dropper can be used to apply one to two drops of blended oils at a time. Oils should be stored with a cap and a dropper should be used exclusively to extract the oil to minimize any contamination. Most oils are so strong they will pull toxins from the plastic dropper, so it is safest to store the oil in glass and only use the dropper for extraction. Rather than using evenly blended oils, single drops of each essential oil can also be used for more intensity or to put more emphasis on specific oils.

Immune System Support

For basic immune system support every day, orange oil and cinnamon oil are a good pairing, with one drop of each or up to two drops maximum of orange oil. This not only provides an uplifting experience but tastes good as well. For an extra immune boost and to target more oral health issues, add one drop of clove oil. This is a very good blend to use for the fall and winter due to its warming properties. It will lessen the occurrence of immune challenges if used during the summer to fall transition.

Dental Infection

1 tablespoon of coconut oil

1 drop each of cinnamon, clove, and lemon essential oils

Immune Support

1 tablespoon of coconut oil

1 drop each of cinnamon, orange, and clove essential oils

Cleansing and Uplifting

A cleansing and disinfecting blend that is light and fruity, yet powerful, is lemon, grapefruit, and orange oils. These oils all focus on supporting different detoxification pathways while also providing a side benefit of lifting you out of a low mood. This would be a good spring and summer blend for seasonal support and would be great to use for the winter to spring season change to help the liver process new pollens and minimize allergies.

Bad Breath

1 tablespoon of coconut oil

1 drop of peppermint oil

Detox Support

1 tablespoon of coconut or sesame oil

1 drop each of lemon, grapefruit, and orange essential oils

Pregnancy Energy Combinations

1 tablespoon of coconut, sesame, or sunflower oil

1 drop of grapefruit, lemon, or orange essential oils

Toothache

1 tablespoon of coconut, sesame, or sunflower oil

1 drop of clove essential oil

Weight Loss

1 tablespoon of coconut oil

1 drop each of grapefruit, lemon, and peppermint essential oils

Sinus Support

According to Chinese medicine, if the sinuses are blocked, that often means the liver needs support. A great blend to help open sinuses is lemon and peppermint. Lemon focuses on body-wide detoxification but also supports the liver, while peppermint supports sinus clearing and helps overall head congestion. This is a good blend to use with headaches and hangovers. The oils would be best blended at a one to one ratio of one or two drops per pulling session.

Headaches or Allergies

1 tablespoon of sesame, coconut, or sunflower oil

1 drop each of peppermint, lemon, and lavender essential oils

Seasonal Change

1 tablespoon of sesame or coconut oil

1 drop each of cinnamon and orange essential oils

Sinus Support

1 tablespoon of coconut oil

1 drop of peppermint essential oil

1 drop of lemon essential oil

Digestive Support

A good blend to support digestion would consist of peppermint, ginger, and fennel. From a flavor perspective, this would be slightly spicy and from a scent perspective, it would be quite uplifting! This blend would greatly support the liver and could be used to support detoxification after overindulging in food or alcohol. This would be best blended on a one to one ratio.

Candida Infection

1 tablespoon of sesame oil

1 drop of oregano essential oil (Oregano oil is VERY STRONG, so the Immune Support recipe on page 84 will also help, but oregano is best for this type of infection.)

Gas and Bloating

1 tablespoon of sesame, sunflower, or coconut oil

1 drop each of peppermint, fennel, and ginger essential oils

Nausea or Pregnancy Morning Sickness

1 tablespoon of coconut oil

1 drop of ginger essential oil

Relaxation or Sleep Support

If pulling before bedtime or with the desired outcome to calm down or supportively uplift mood in an unstimulating way, lavender and bergamot are a great blend. A one to one ratio should be used.

Lavender used alone is calming, but if a bit more support is needed, the hormones will be more supported by the bergamot.

Fatigue

1 tablespoon of sesame, sunflower, or coconut oil

1 drop each of lemon and peppermint essential oils

Insomnia (to use at night)

1 tablespoon of coconut oil

1 drop each of bergamot and lavender essential oils

CHAPTER 7

WORKING OIL PULLING INTO YOUR LIFE

Where Can You Fit This New Oil-Pulling Habit?

Now that you know all of the amazing reasons why oil pulling should be a part of your life—whiter teeth, healthier gums, fewer cavities, clearer sinuses, better skin, fewer headaches, a cleaner liver, improved digestion, a healthier heart, and a better immune system—how do you fit this amazing and necessary habit into an already bustling schedule?

It really all comes down to logistics, planning, and figuring out what works best for you, then making it a healthy habit. This can sound WAY more intimidating than it really is. It is possible to get you and those you love doing this life-changing, health-advancing, money-saving habit!

First step to making this routine a part of your life is to make friends with an oil you like. The best way to do this is to choose one and start there. After everything you have read so far, is there an oil that sounds like one you would not mind spending 20 minutes a day being good friends with? Sometimes you can even approach it from a taste preference. Does coconut or sesame sound good to you? Those are the most common, so that is a good starting point. Then, you need to get a high-quality oil. There are quite a few resources online to buy quality oils from and most health food stores or specialty grocery stores also sell high-quality oils.

Oil storage is an important point to cover. Oils are best stored in a glass container. This is why, as you may notice, most oils are actually sold in a glass container. Another thing that is important is to keep the oils in a safe place away from sunlight. Oils can change or oxidize if exposed to too much light, and this will change the benefits you may receive from them. Another point on oil storage is to keep the container small. If you buy in bulk, transfer some of the oil to a smaller container for daily opening. If you open a big container every day, more and more air will get into the container, compromising the quality of the oil. You want to keep your oil as fresh as possible and this includes protecting it from the elements.

Where you keep your oil may help encourage the habit. Many people just forget to oil pull or find going to the kitchen to grab the oil time-consuming or inconvenient. Keeping a jar of oil and a spoon in your bathroom may seem too weird for some people. If the medicine cabinet or cabinet under the sink is too weird, find a safe, dark place in your bedroom that seems to make more sense to you. Most people keep their toothbrushes in their bathroom; oil and a spoon are no different, really.

When to Oil Pull

A great way to work oil pulling in first thing in the morning is to pull in the shower. It is a good 15 to 20 minutes from stepping in the shower to toweling off and getting dressed. Why not swish the whole time?

Another great option timewise is to get up a bit early and check emails or social media while you are pulling. The only caution here is to avoid coming across something too emotional or too funny! If you start to laugh you could end up spitting your oil out, and that would be a mess to clean up.

Another potentially messy situation is sneezing. If you feel a sneeze coming on, spit the oil out into a cup or the trash. This sounds pretty straightforward, but your instincts may sometimes have you do the opposite and you could end up hurting yourself in the process of trying to keep it in, straining your neck or inhaling or swallowing bacteria-filled oil! And NOBODY wants to end up with oil up their nose, but that is obviously a worst-case scenario.

Getting your loved ones on board with oil pulling is a wonderful idea. Get the kids to do it too! It is possible, and there are moms everywhere reporting wins on cavities with oil pulling. The key is to make it fun or to incentivize doing it. Not getting cavities may not even be a good enough reason for an adult to do it, so it needs to be decided what the motivating factor will be. For many adults and teens, the teeth-whitening benefits for such a reasonable price is a great starting point! Better breath is also a good one. Nobody wants stinky breath!

For kids, the benefits might be having to brush less and decreasing the amount of time needed for brushing. Kids can join the whole family for a morning oil-pulling session. A great way to get kids to do it is to let them choose a flavor of essential oil they can add into the base oil. Also, have them work up to 20 minutes, rewarding them with stars on a chart every time they move up in time. After that, you can have them earn stars for each time they pull for a certain amount of time, and you can give them a healthy treat for each time they get 5 to 10 stars. From a dental health perspective, this habit is far better than sending the kids down the route toward cavities and, someday, root canals.

Traveling while oil pulling is also easy to do! At most health food stores, very small bottles or packets of oils are available for purchase. In the coconut oil section you can often find smaller-sized bottles more fit for travel.

The other possibility is to grab a small, used glass jar. You can clean it well then add your coconut or sesame oil and even blend your essential oil into the base oil for ease while traveling. You can actually blend the oils at home, too, if you decide on an essential oil that makes sense to pull with above all others. The main thing to note is once an essential oil is chosen, it must only be stored in glass. If you put it in plastic, the essential oil might leach the plastic into the oil mixture.

Oil pulling fits in so easily to a healthy lifestyle because you likely already have oils as a part of your life.

Troubleshooting
Face, Neck, and Jaw Pain

Some of the main issues or problems that people report while oil pulling are jaw soreness, fatigue, and even facial pain. These are usually signs that you are swishing the oil too vigorously. You want to move the oil about the mouth and in between the teeth, but not so much that the 20 minutes is exhausting and you are left with face, neck, or jaw pain.

Tension Headaches

People have also reported tension headaches from pulling. This could be due to excessive motion, as just discussed, or even the need to scale back and work up to a 20-minute pulling session. You can pull for 5 minutes the first week then increase by 5 minutes per week until you are at 20 minutes of pulling per session. Another possibility is that you have a problem with your TMJ, or jaw joint. This can be best evaluated by a dentist who specializes in TMJ issues. Sometimes, a certain activity like this can bring your attention to an issue. It does not mean you cannot oil pull, it just means you may need some additional support so you can do this every day. If this is your situation, please do not stop the oil pulling. Get the TMJ problem handled, as it would have become symptomatic someday anyway. Find out what is needed to support your TMJ, then get back to your daily oil-pulling routine!

Gagging

Gagging can be another issue when you oil pull. This one can be fairly common when you first start. Most often, the same gentle time schedule of 5 minutes for a week with a 5-minute increase per week until you reach 20 minutes per day resolves the problem. The other fix is to really make sure you are not letting the oil get too far back into the throat. Adding ginger or peppermint essential oil to the base oil can help as well. Finally, try less oil. Sometimes people produce a lot of saliva in response to the oil, so that can be overwhelming to the mouth and throat and end up eliciting a gag response. Some people just gag easily. You may have to experiment to see if there is some other variable that might help, like not moving or keeping the head in a certain position. Another possibility is that certain body systems, like the digestive system, liver, or gallbladder, need support. Seeing a health care practitioner that specializes in nutrition or herbal medicine is a good idea.

Stuffy Nose

A severely stuffed-up nose can stop the pulling process due to the need to breathe. Inhaling some peppermint or eucalyptus oil can help open sinuses. Or, use a Neti pot or sinus rinse squeeze bottle before you pull to clear the sinuses.

Some people begin to stuff up while pulling. This is actually a good sign, as it is the body's way of preparing to get rid of bacteria. The only challenge, again, is breathing. If it is not too severe, continuing to oil pull should help to stop the issue. However, it may be necessary to stop, clear the passages, and start over.

Again, adding peppermint essential oil to the base oil will also help to open sinuses.

Some people notice that oil pulling in a steamy shower helps to handle a lot of potential problems, this one especially.

How Healthy Should You Be to Pull?

Optimally you would be feeling pretty good when you oil pull in case it does bring on a healing crisis (page 33). Some people, however, report that oil pulling through a sickness helps them feel better. Since it activates cleansing and detoxification, it can be helpful. Again, this is really based on the individual. Ideally, embarking on oil pulling gets you back to a better state of health, so stay proactive and do it daily!

Staying Hydrated

You have probably heard that our bodies consist primarily of water. One of the most important things that can be done to support the body's detoxification is to drink water. This helps the liver to filter any toxins, and is needed for optimal kidney function as well. If you consume enough water, you can eradicate body odor or greatly dissipate it to the point where you'll no longer need deodorants. The sweat will become more clear and pure in nature, as toxins are more easily expelled. A good rule of thumb is to drink eight or more glasses a day, depending on the weather and your activity level. If you are in a hot climate, sit in a sauna daily, or have a disciplined workout routine, then you would need more than eight glasses. If you live in a cold, snowy climate and are fairly inactive, you would need less. A good sign you are getting adequate water is producing urine with a pale, light yellow color.

Adequate Rest

Our crazy-busy, stressful lives leave us with little downtime. Improving your health via detoxification requires extra energy of your bodily systems. It should not leave you exhausted; however, you will need adequate sleep and rest for your body to handle all of the things needed to detoxify properly. A minimum of seven hours of sleep a night is recommended to get the full benefits from your oil-pulling habit.

A Healthy Diet

The Standard American Diet, or "SAD," includes items that are not good at all for dental and oral health and happen to negatively impact the entire body. The "SAD" diet includes processed foods, especially those high in starch and sugar, and foods that include partially hydrogenated fats. Most of the "SAD" foods are found by shopping the middle of the grocery store where food is in boxes. Now let's be honest, you can eat whatever you want and still get benefits from oil pulling. If you are reading this, though, you are likely already interested in improving your health.

So what are the best foods for that? The field of nutrition and diet has changed a lot over the years, making it challenging to know what kinds of foods to eat. We have come a long way from the food pyramid many know so well.

The work of dentist Weston A. Price holds compelling evidence as to how we should approach eating. During his travels, he found that the people who had little to no degenerative diseases, cancers, debility, or endocrine disorders and had BEAUTIFUL MOUTHS AND TEETH lived in areas without modern-day processed foods. Though these societies were remote, the tribes living within them ate healthier foods than most Americans do today with the "SAD." These people were eating animals, fish, veggies, nuts, legumes, and whole grains. The bottom line is they were eating real food, including quality protein sources and high amounts of plant-based foods. They were also eating quality fats. Eating thusly nourishes the whole body while creating a healthy environment for the mouth and gums. Oil pulling should become a frequent habit, but it helps to have fewer projects to combat while doing it! Eating starchy and/or sugary foods creates a breeding ground for organisms that just want to eat away at teeth and gums and cause problems.

Certain foods are actually considered beneficial to oral health and should be included in your diet. One of the best-known dental issues more prevalent today than most would think is scurvy, caused by a lack of vitamin C. With this disease, the gums rot away and the teeth are in danger of falling out. Vitamin C in citrus fruits is utilized by the body much more readily than that from a vitamin C tablet. Berries are another food that should be consumed. They contain anthocyanins necessary for tissue healing and strength of blood vessel walls. All of those tiny capillaries at the base of the teeth need as much support as they can get. Bone broth has recently come back into favor. In China, when someone is really ill, they're given bone broth daily until they can stomach more foods. This is the most nourishing food on the planet! Bone broth actually contains the trace minerals needed to build healthy bones, thus supporting your jaw to help build healthy teeth. The calcium in bone broth is the most easily absorbed by the human body. In many cultures around the world, this is a staple. In the "SAD" diet, it has been replaced by store-bought, boxed broth with little benefit. Many recipes found in books and online can show you how to make it. Paleo books are a good reference for this.

Fermented foods are a great way to introduce healthy bacteria into the body. The most common fermented foods are sauerkraut, kim chi, miso, tempeh, yogurt, and kefir. The most common fermented drinks are kombucha tea and lassi. There are lots of books on how to make your own, but all of these items are easily found at health food stores. By introducing good bacteria into the mouth and digestive tract, you balance the system against bad bacteria.

Daily Exercise

One of the most interesting things about the human body is that we are covered in this intricate system for detoxification called the lymphatic system. Most of you know you have lymph nodes because when you were sick as a child, sometimes they would swell up and your mom, dad, or the doctor would feel the slightly puffy, sore area on your neck. That soreness was due to your lymph node collecting the bacteria that your body was killing and expelling from the body. This system can be found throughout your entire body. You can actually outline the human body in lymph nodes and see the shape of the arms, legs, torso, and head!

The thing about this system is it requires movement to pump toxins through the chain of lymph nodes throughout your body. When you get up and exercise, you greatly enhance the function of your lymphatic system.

Oil pulling benefits can be greatly enhanced by a daily exercise regimen. Walking for 30 minutes multiple times a week should suffice. It is well-documented, however, that yoga is a great way to reach even deeper levels of lymphatic drainage and movement. Exercise greatly enhances how your whole body functions, from the cardiovascular system, lungs, and kidneys to the nervous system, immune system, and more. Overall, it should be a huge part of your oil-pulling lifestyle.

Sauna, Massage, and Hot Baths

Saunas and massages are two wonderful ways to help the body detoxify and drain. Heating up the body tissues and sweating activate more detoxification pathways. Once you start oil pulling, it opens the body to doing this kind of work by wanting to expel toxins.

A dry, hot sauna is a wonderful way to liberate some of those toxins stored deep in your body tissues. Some people even like oil pulling in the sauna! Depending on the type, you are generally in the sauna for 5 to 20 minutes, which is the perfect amount of time for oil pulling as well!

A great way to move the lymphatic system for someone who may be in poorer health or who cannot exercise is massage. Massage is a wonderful, passive bodywork activity that is very encouraging to the circulation of the entire body while promoting the detoxification of all systems. A great time to oil pull would be after a massage. The stomach will more likely be on the emptier side after a 60 to 90 minute session, and you can throw in a quick 5 to 20 minutes of oil pulling to help the body expel any toxins released. Don't forget to rehydrate with water before or after oil pulling to help the kidneys get rid of any toxins they can remove.

Taking a nice, hot bath quickly and easily heats up the deep tissues, which will start to release so toxins that can be removed by the body via the detoxification pathways. Oil pulling can assist this process and is also easily done in the bath for the 5- to 20-minute duration.

The Ayurvedic Lifestyle

After delving into this wonderful habit you might wonder what else you can do to support your body. There is lots of information available about the health system that introduced oil pulling to the world. Learning about what dosha (page 18) or body type you are can lead you to more specific clues about which herbs and foods your body might prefer, what oils might work best, and which exercises to choose. Incorporating these principles along with clean eating by avoiding the "SAD" diet foods and a diet based on real food will help you live a healthier, happier life!

Oil Pulling for Kids

Oil pulling is a safe and healthy habit for kids to do. So many kids end up with cavities and have to go through the painstaking process of visiting the dentist for treatment. Many families have reported great success teaching kids as young as four how to oil pull. Have them start with a smaller amount of oil and teach them to swish it around without swallowing.

Coconut oil is great to use with kids. They tend to think it is funny because it usually starts out more solid and turns liquid while swishing. Kids should pull for a maximum of 5 to 10 minutes. They do not have the same amount of toxins that adults do. When kids get into their teen years, they can also pull for 20 minutes. I have a patient that made oil pulling a family affair when her daughter was getting frequent cavities at age seven. After oil pulling for two months almost daily, the dentist reevaluated the girl. She no longer needed any fillings and had fewer cavities.

Oil Pulling for Animals

Okay, okay...so you cannot teach your pet to oil pull. After reading all of this, though, you cannot be blamed if it crossed your mind! Of course you want what's best for your animal! While you cannot teach them to oil pull, you can, however, use oil to help their oral health. One of the things you can do is to brush their teeth over and over with oil. They will ingest the oil, so pick one that is safe for your pet and make sure you are not going to be at risk of getting bitten! Also, you can make coconut oil chews in the freezer as discussed earlier. Dogs love coconut oil, which they can chew and ingest. The coconut oil is said to boost their immune system, freshen their breath, and help with many other potential issues that pets encounter.

The thing about animals' bodies is they have really strong stomach acid to break down any bacteria they encounter. They will just excrete it through their digestive tracts.

CONCLUSION

Every day we can read health-related news in a newspaper, a magazine, or the Internet. Oftentimes, we learn new things or find we must unlearn something we once thought was healthy. What I've recently discovered is that the roots of health tend to be found in older traditions exercised by our ancestors. Some of the simplest things, like gargling with lemon and honey in hot water, can help a cough and sore throat. Among all the expensive dental care products and fancy, processed foods that exist on the market, getting back to basics is not only cost-effective, it works!

If you want whiter teeth but prefer to avoid expensive and potentially toxic remedies sold in the store, try oil pulling! If you want to skirt buying a jug of mouthwash that could potentially add more toxins to your system, try oil pulling! After doing a cost-benefit analysis, you will find it is worth your time and money to add this habit to your life. I guarantee you will be hooked very soon after noticing how your teeth feel instantly smoother. There are many compelling case reports of success for many different health reasons and so much science behind why this habit is good for you. They make it hard to believe you wouldn't be compelled to try it.

Remember, give oil pulling sufficient time before judging what it is doing for you. As a practitioner, I've learned our society expects quick results. I think it is great to think like an optimist! I have learned, however, that healing does take time. You will likely see some quick results, but continue to spend a few months with this wonderful healthy habit and watch it improve your life one day at a time.

REFERENCES

AromaTools. *Modern Essentials: A Contemporary Guide to the Therapeutic Use of Essential Oils, 5th Edition.* Orem, UT: AromaTools, 2014.

Asokan et al. 2011. "Effect of Oil Pulling on Halitosis and Microorganisms Causing Halitosis: A Randomized Controlled Pilot Trail." *Journal of Indian Society of Pedodontics and Preventive Dentistry* 29(2): 90–94.

Asokan et al. 2009. "Effect of Oil Pulling on Plaque-Induced Gingivitis: A Randomized, Controlled, Triple-Blind Study." *Indian Journal of Dental Research* 20(1): 47–51.

Asokan et al. March 2008. "Effect of Oil Pulling on Streptococcus Mutans Count in Plaque and Saliva Using Dentocult SM Strip Mutans Test: A Randomized, Controlled, Triple-Blind Study." *Journal of Indian Society of Pedadontics and Preventive Dentistry* 26(1): 12–17.

Asokan et al. 2011. "Mechanism of Oil-Pulling Therapy—In Vitro Study." *Indian Journal of Dental Research* 22(1): 34–37.

Cheshire, Sara. August 6, 2014. "Does Oil Pulling Work?" http://www.cnn.com/2014/08/06/health/oil-pulling/index.html.

Doheny, Kathleen. March 10, 2008. "Drugs in Our Drinking Water?" www.webmd.com/a-to-z-guides/features/drugs-in-our-drinking-water.

Lad, Vasant. *The Complete Book of Ayurvedic Home Remedies*. New York: Three Rivers Press, 1999.

Larsen, Sonja. *The Beauty Books: Oil Pulling for Cleansing, Healing and Feeling Alive*. Los Angeles: Blue Sun Media, 2014.

Mercola. May 5, 2014. "Oil Pulling Craze: All-Purpose Remedy?" http://articles.mercola.com/sites/articles/archive/2014/05/05/oil-pulling-coconut-oil.aspx.

Narasimhulu et al. 2015. "Anti-atherosclerotic and Anti-inflammatory Actions of Sesame Oil." *Journal of Medicinal Food* 18(1):11–20.

Oakley, Colleen. June 4, 2014. "Should You Try Oil Pulling?" http://www.webmd.com/oral-health/features/oil-pulling.

Ogawa, Nishio, and Okada. September 2013. "Effect of Edible Sesame Oil on Growth of Clinical Isolates of Candida Albicans." *Biological Research for Nursing* 16(3): 335–43.

Rogers, Sherry. *Detoxify or Die*. Sarasota, FL: SandKey Company, 2002.

Saleem, Chetty, and Kavimani. September 2013. "Putative Antioxidant Property of Sesame Oil in an Oxidative Stress Model of Myocardial Injury." *Journal of Cardiovascular Disease Research* 4(3): 177–81.

Singh and Purohit. April 2011. "Tooth Brushing, Oil Pulling and Tissue Regeneration: A Review of Holistic Approaches to Oral Health." *Journal of Ayurveda and Integrative Medicine* 2(2): 64–68.

Sood et al. November 2014. "Comparative Efficacy of Oil Pulling and Chlorhexidine on Malodor: A Randomized Controlled Trail." *Journal of Clinical and Diagnostic Research* 8(11): ZC18–21.

Weston A. Price Foundation website, accessed January 17, 2015. http://www.westonaprice.org/.

Worwood, Valerie Ann. *The Complete Book of Essential Oils and Aromatherapy*. Novato, CA: New World Library, 1991.

INDEX

ACKNOWLEDGMENTS

I would like to acknowledge the two people who encouraged me to begin sharing my knowledge through the written word: Dr. Lauren Clum and Dr. Mariza Snyder. I would like to thank my patients for putting up with a very busy doctor while I was busy writing parts of this book. I would like to acknowledge Dr. Preet Sahota for inspiring me to look at dental health from a holistic perspective. I would like to acknowledge my parents, John and Debbie, for always encouraging me to chase after my dreams of entrepreneurship. I would like to thank my husband, Erick, for always believing in me and for inspiring me to grow.

ABOUT THE AUTHOR

Dr. Michelle Coleman is a chiropractor and nutritionist and the owner of Bella Wellness Center, a multidisciplinary health clinic in Danville, California, that offers nutrition, chiropractic, acupuncture, and massage services. She has been in private practice for the past decade and supports many of her professional associations. She is happily married to a successful chiropractor and is a loving stepmother to three very healthy and active children. Her main passions outside work are being active, cooking healthy, and constantly striving to make her community a healthier and happier place to live.